Neurology in General Practice

Neurology in General Practice

G David Perkin FRCP
Consultant Neurologist,
West London Neurosciences Centre,
Charing Cross Hospital,
London, UK

MARTIN DUNITZ

© 2002 Martin Dunitz Ltd, a member of the Taylor & Francis group

First published in the United Kingdom in 2002 by Martin Dunitz Ltd
The Livery House, 7–9 Pratt Street, London NW1 0AE

Tel: +44 (0)20 7482 2202
Fax: +44 (0)20 7267 0159
E-mail: info.dunitz@tandf.co.uk
Website: http://www.dunitz.co.uk

A CIP record for this book is available from the British Library

ISBN 1-84184-039-4

Distributed in the USA by
Fulfilment Center
Taylor & Francis
7625 Empire Drive
Florence, KY 41042, USA
Toll Free Tel: 1-800-634-7064
Email: cserve@routledge_ny.com

Distributed in Canada by
Taylor & Francis
74 Rolark Drive
Scarborough
Ontario M1R 4G2, Canada
Toll Free Tel: 1-877-226-2237
Email: tal_fran@istar.ca

Distributed in the rest of the world by
ITPS Limited
Cheriton House
North Way, Andover
Hampshire SP10 5BE, UK
Tel: +44 (0) 1264 332424
Email: reception@itps.co.uk

Printed and bound in Italy by Printer trento S.r.l.

Contents

Introduction

Data on the contribution of neurological disorders to the general practitioner's workload have come from a number of sources. Surveys of specific neurological conditions or symptoms from individual practices have been performed – for example the distribution of headache type in patients complaining of headache as their principal symptom.[1] More comprehensive material has emerged from investigators (most conspicuously, perhaps John Fry) who collected data on the distribution of disease among general practice referrals over many years. In Fry's last contribution to this literature (Table 1) a breakdown of neurological disease in terms of its likely presentation to a general practitioner, according to practice size, was summarized.[2]

The value of such data is inevitably dependent on the criteria used for making individual diagnoses. A more recent publication has addressed this issue, and in doing so has provided the most accurate current data on the incidence and lifetime prevalence of neurological disorders as ascertained from general practice and subsequently appraised by specialist opinion.[3] Six per cent of the population studied (totalling 100,230 patients) had had a neurological disorder at some time. Age- and sex-adjusted rates for the more common neurological disorders (Table 2) were generally similar to rates reported from previous surveys.

Disease	Persons Consulting Annually	
	Per 2000	Per 10 000
Stroke	12	60
(Acute stroke)	6	30
Transient ischaemic attack (TIA)	4	20
Migraine	16	80
Headache	34	170
Dizziness, vertigo	30	150
Epilepsy	12	60
Syncope (faint)	8	40
Parkinsonism	4	20
Multiple Sclerosis	2	10
Brain tumour	(1 in 10 years)	(1 in 2 years)
Motor neurone disease	(1 in 20 years)	(1 in 4 years)
Meningitis	(1 in 5 years)	(1 yearly)

Adapted from Fry and Sandler,[2] with kind permission of Kluwer Academic Publishers.

Table 1
Annual consultation rates for neurological disorders

(Conspicuous absentees from the list, including migraine, tension headache and carpal tunnel syndrome, were not ascertained because of the study's resource constraints.) The figures correspond reasonably closely to Fry's data. Inevitably, such prevalence figures are matched by the distribution of neurological disorders seen in a general neurology outpatient setting (Table 3.)[4]

Neurological disorders, therefore, represent a significant component of a general practitioner's workload. Including eye and ear complaints they account for 13% of all consultations.[5]

Condition	Age and sex-adjusted rate (95% CI), 100,000 per year
Stroke:	
First cerebrovascular episode	205
Second cerebrovascular episode	42
Intracranial haemorrhage	10
Epilepsy:	46
Single seizures	11
Primary neurological CNS tumours (benign and malignant)	10
Parkinson's disease	19
Compressive neuropathies (except carpal tunnel syndrome)	49

Adapted from MacDonald et al,[3] with kind permission of OUP.

Table 2
Age and sex-adjusted rates for common neurological conditions

The following chapters deal first with common neurological complaints and how they are best managed at an initial consultation and then cover management issues of specific neurological disorders in the general practice setting. A recurring theme in these chapters is the need for general practice to take on a higher profile in patients with neurological disease, both in terms of initial assessment and recognition and also in terms of ongoing support for those patients (and their carers) who have chronic neurological disease.

Nurse practitioners with experience in a particular condition are becoming the norm in hospital practice. There are nurses with a special interest in multiple sclerosis, epilepsy, stroke and Parkinson's disease, and these nurses function largely through the hospital service. An expansion

		%
No diagnosis	2075	26.5
Epilepsy	813	10.4
Tension headache	589	7.5
Cerebrovascular disease	576	7.4
Migraine	389	5.0
Entrapment neuropathy	345	4.4
Conversion hysteria	297	3.8
Anatomical	290	3.7
Multiple sclerosis	274	3.5
Vasovagal	163	2.1
Hyperventilation	159	2.0
Parkinson's disease	149	1.9
Post-traumatic syndrome	139	1.8
Dementia	121	1.5
Peripheral neuropathy	107	1.4
Depression	106	1.4
Non-neurological diagnosis	103	1.3
Cervical radiculopathy/myelopathy	94	1.2
Lumbar spondylosis	77	1.0
Essential tremor	74	0.9

Adapted from Perkin,[4] with kind permission of the BMJ Publishing Group.

Table 3
Top 20 diagnoses among 7836 successive neurology outpatient referrals

of their role, leading to their working in general practices, would allow an expansion of care within general practice and heighten awareness of particular neurological conditions.[6]

Would unfettered access to diagnostic services enhance the general practitioner's role, or would it simply flood the system with unwarranted requests? A pilot study of 100 MRI requests from a group of practices in Lothian (all vetted by a consultant neuroradiologist) produced the same yield of abnormal scans that were considered to be radiologically significant as a comparable number of scan requests emanating from hospital clinicians. This study was preceded by a workshop for general practitioners on the use of magnetic resonance imaging (MRI); nevertheless, it suggests that direct access to certain services might enhance general practice care without distorting the function of the relevant department.

Common problems in general practice

The commonest symptoms encountered in neurological practice are headache, dizziness, altered sensations and episodes of altered awareness. Perhaps 20 per cent of patients presenting with such symptoms remain undiagnosed, the percentage almost certainly rising for these patients who present with the same symptoms in general practice. Lists of underlying conditions which have to be considered in such patients, therefore, need to take account of such diagnostic uncertainty.

Headache

Causes of headache include:

- tension headache;

- migraine;

- cervical spondylosis;

- temporomandibular joint dysfunction;

- cerebral tumour;

- meningitis;

- subarachnoid haemorrhage;

- cranial arteritis.

Too often, patients with headache are referred from general practice to a neurologist on the assumption (frequently specifically requested) that investigation is necessary for the diagnosis. Nothing is further from the truth. Patients with chronic headache, whether recurrent or persistent are diagnosed on the basis of their history, not on investigation. Most headache and facial pain syndromes are stereotypical (eg trigeminal neuralgia, cranial arteritis) and though investigation may be valuable as a confirmatory measure (an elevated ESR and an abnormal temporal artery biopsy in cranial arteritis, for example) they supplement rather than replace accurate history taking.

Acute headache is a different situation and may demand urgent hospital referral if there is a suspicion of meningeal irritation.

Dizziness

Lists of causes of dizziness presuppose that the complaint is sufficiently specific to allow accurate diagnosis. The complaint means different things to different patients (and doctors) necessitating therefore that, where possible, further definition of the symptom is attempted. Vertigo is not a diagnosis, but merely another symptom, implying a sense of rotation of the self or of the environment.

Causes of dizziness include:

- benign positional vertigo;

- acute labyrinthitis;

- anxiety state;

- hyperventilation syndrome;

- brain stem vascular or demyelinating disease.

The value of the history is in establishing the mode of onset of the symptom, its triggering factors (if any) and the environments in which it occurs. Benign positional vertigo classically occurs when the patient turns over in bed. Acute labyrinthitis is of acute onset, with prominent vertigo and ataxia, coupled with nausea, vomiting and malaise.The condition is self-limiting. The dizziness of an anxiety state, or of hyperventilation often occurs in particular environments, eg supermarkets. If these connections are not appreciated, and therefore not enquired after, diagnoses will remain undiscovered.

Altered sensations

Patients often use medical terms in different ways from their doctors. Numbness is a case in point. To a doctor, the term should mean some impairment of cutaneous sensation. If that is not the patient's complaint, the term should not be used. With increasing Internet access, patients are frequently scanning the Internet for an explanation for their complaint, prior to consultation with the doctor. Fears of particular conditions are raised, for example multiple sclerosis, which will not be allayed, rather reinforced, by wholesale referral to a neurologist. Better to establish the nature of the patient's complaint, its distribution and its time course as a way of better understanding its causation.

Causes of altered sensations include:

- mononeuropathies (eg carpal tunnel syndrome);

- radiculopathies;

- cervical myelopathy;

- cerebrovascular disease.

Many patients with sensory symptoms have very nebulous complaints which are difficult to relate to a particular part of the nervous system. Such patients can be reasonably reviewed in the practice after an interval to determine whether more specific problems have arisen.

Altered awareness

It is vital, when doctors see patients with episodes of altered awareness, that an eye witness account, if available, is obtained and, ideally, that the eyewitness accompanies the patient. Though epilepsy is common, so are vasovagal attacks. The distinction is not always easy, but is certainly facilitated by an accurate history.

Causes of altered awareness include:

- vasovagal attacks (simple faints);

- epilepsy;

- situational syncope (eg during micturition);

- cardiac syncope.

The age of the patient is of importance. Older patients may appear to 'faint' but such episodes are commonly triggered either by postural hypotension or by a cardiac arrhythmia. Drug enquiry is vital in such patients.

Other neurological presentations and questions to ask are summarised in Table 4.

Complaint	Important questions	Conditions to consider
Loss of vision	1. Unilateral or bilateral 2. Distribution of vision loss 3. Mode of onset 4. Ocular pain	Optic neuritis Retinal detachment Retinal vascular accident Stroke
Diplopia	1. In which direction of gaze 2. Vertical or horizontal separation 3. Other symptoms 4. Fatiguability	Brain stem CVA 'Arteriosclerotic' Myasthenia Multiple sclerosis
Dysarthria	1. Just articulation problem or speech content disorder also 2. Other symptoms 3. Swallow problems	CVA Multiple sclerosis Myasthenia Motor neuron disease
Weakness	1. Distribution 2. Mode of onset 3. Fatiguability 4. Previous episodes	CVA Multiple sclerosis Peripheral neuropathy Myasthenia Motor neuron disease
Loss of memory	1. Duration 2. Mode of onset 3. Apparent to patient 4. Stress factors	Dementia Anxiety state Depressive illness
Altered gait	1. Deviating to one side 2. Slowness of initiation 3. Dragging one or both legs 4. Catching feet	CVA Peripheral neuropathy Parkinson's disease Multiple sclerosis Cerebellar disorders

Table 4
Neurological presentations and questions to ask

Investigation

Plain x-rays

Of very limited value. Skull x-rays are of no value other than in trauma. Plain x-rays of the spine are usually abnormal in individuals over the age of 50.

CT scanning

A very valuable investigation which can be performed rapidly. Liable to abuse however. The vast majority of patients with headache don't need one. Restricted access for many general practitioners.

MR Scanning

Highly sophisticated and very informative imaging system. Frequently detects non-specific signal change in the brain, particularly in those over 40. Best used in conjunction with neurological advice.

EMG

A very valuable technique for the investigation of peripheral nerve and muscle disease. Crucially dependent on the quality of the electrophysiologist.

EEG

A valuable test in the assessment of possible epilepsy. However many patients with epilepsy have a normal EEG.

CSF

Used increasingly less often. Invaluable for the assessment of suspected meningitis and subarachnoid haemorrhage. Otherwise, its main value is for the assessment of multiple sclerosis, though that indication is receding.

Psychometry

Allows a formal appraisal of an individual's intellectual function and whether it has altered as a result of a disease process. Essential for the appraisal of suspected dementia. Very often serves to establish that a complaint of memory loss has been triggered by psychological factors. The procedure is usually arranged through a hospital referral.

Headache

Epidemiology

Since headache is an almost universal experience (80–90 per cent of the population have experienced a headache at some time in the previous 12 months), it is perhaps surprising that headache is not more conspicuous in the list of complaints leading to consultation with the general practitioner. In the USA, it has been calculated that 4.3 annual visits per 100 of the population are due to headache. In a UK survey, headache was the predominant complaint in both 4 per cent of consecutive practice consultations and home visits.[8] Analysis of the underlying diagnosis is critically dependent on the criteria used for those diagnoses. In one survey of 200 successive headache patients encountered in general practice, migraine and tension headache accounted for the majority (66.5 per cent) (Table 5).[1] This 66.5 per cent of the total is very close to the 58.6 per cent that migraine and tension headache contribute to the headaches seen in neurological practice.[4] The major difference between general and neurological practice in terms of causes of headache relates to headache attributable to an infective illness – a rarity in neurological practice, it accounted for 42 per cent of the patients in Milne's series,[8] rising to over 90 per cent for people at home.

Cause	Number of patients	Percentage
Tension headache	74	37
Migraine	59	29.5
Fevers	20	10
Sinus	11	5.5
Hypertension	10	5.0
Cervical arthritis	5	2.5
Post-traumatic	5	2.5
Others	16	8
Adapted from Jerrett.[1]		

Table 5
Classification of the cause of headache in 200 patients

Important features in the history

A histogram of headache type according to time course and severity is shown in Figure 1.

Duration of history

Brain tumour is rarely encountered in general practice, and seldom, if ever, does the patient present with headache alone. The duration of the history is of critical importance. Around half the patients with migraine or tension headache who are seen in neurology outpatient departments have a history of longer than 1 year.

Patients often forget their previous complaints. Careful practice records will ensure that, if there is a longer history of headache, it has been previously documented. A new headache, therefore, particularly in an older person, is a potential cause of concern.

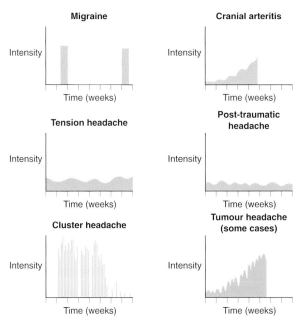

Figure 1
Headache type according to time course and severity

Distribution of headache

The distribution of headache is seldom helpful in making a diagnosis. Many migraine headaches are diffuse rather than unilateral. Most tension headaches (and non-specific headaches) are bilateral. Tumour headaches and headaches related to cranial arteritis can be either focal or diffuse.

Quality and severity of headache

Again, neither the quality nor the severity of headache is necessarily helpful. Many patients with cerebral tumours have mild or negligible headache. Cluster headache is far more severe than most tumour headache. Stabbing, pressure, band-like or vice-like pains are particularly suggestive of tension headache. Severity of headache is inevitably subjective.

Precipitating factors

Migraine and the headache of brain tumour are typically worsened by exertion, coughing or sneezing. The headache of cranial arteritis is typically worsened by exposure to cold. Cluster headache is very often precipitated by alcohol. Orgasmic headache occurs at orgasm and is usually found in patients with a previous or subsequent history of migraine.

Accompanying physical signs

The only physical sign compatible with tension headache is scalp tenderness. The scalp tenderness of temporal arteritis is focal, with thickening and reduced pulsation of the superficial temporal artery. Focal neurological deficit is compatible with a diagnosis of migraine but only if found during the acute attack. Autonomic symptoms accompanying an attack of cluster headache include unilateral lachrymation, nasal discharge and redness of the eye. Sometimes a Horner's syndrome occurs.

Intercurrent infection

A relationship between headache and chronic sinus disease is at best dubious. Acute sinusitis causing headache is likely to be associated with purulent nasal discharge (if the maxillary sinus is affected) and focal sinus tenderness. The relevant sinus is likely to be opaque or to contain a fluid level on sinus X-ray, although these changes can be evident in asymptomatic people.

A diagnosis of meningitis is strongly suggested by the presence of signs of meningeal irritation (neck stiffness and a positive Kernig's sign), although these signs may not be conspicuous in infants and in the elderly.

| Tension headache |
| Migraine |
| Infective illnesses |
| Oromandibular joint dysfunction |
| Cervical-related headache |
| Tumour (rarely) |
| Cranial arteritis (rarely) |

Table 6
Conditions to consider as causes of headache

Clinical scenarios

Conditions to consider in a patient with headache are listed in Table 6.

Acute isolated headache

The commonest cause of an acute, isolated headache in general practice is an infective process, usually a non-specific viral illness. Meningism with febrile illness is common in childhood, but the possibility of a meningeal illness demands immediate referral. Subarachnoid haemorrhage is rarely seen in general practice (nine cases during 18 years in one series).[8] Meningeal irritation again demands immediate referral. In Fry's series,[2] a practice of 2000 patients was estimated to see one case of meningitis every 5 years. Viral meningitis is more common than bacterial meningitis. Most cases of viral meningitis occur in children and young adults and predominate in the summer and autumn. Although the individual may be lethargic and irritable, their conscious state is normal. Focal neurological signs will be absent other than those reflecting meningeal irritation. Those signs may be inconspicuous in the very young (or the elderly). Rashes can occur with viral meningitis but do not have the purpuric elements associated with meningococcal meningitis. The outcome for bacterial meningitis is worse for children under the age of 1, and for adults over the age of 40. Perhaps surprisingly, duration of illness prior to the recognition of the diagnosis does not correlate with outcome, though the conscious state does. Meningococcal meningitis typically occurs in epidemics. Typical features include headache (which is severe), vomiting, fever, a depressed conscious level and signs of meningeal irritation. The onset may be over hours, or more gradual. The presence of a rash suggests meningococcal septicaemia but can occur with other bacterial agents and with viral meningitis. Administration of intravenous benzylpenicillin to suspected cases of meningococcal meningitis, particularly if there is a haemorrhagic rash, substantially reduces mortality in children, particularly those who are seriously ill. Suitable doses for an adult are 1.2g, for an infant 300mg, and for a child of 1 to 9 years, 600mg. For those with penicillin allergy, cefotaxime is an alternative.

Inevitably, some patients are encountered with their first attack of migraine or cluster headache. A history of migraine in a family member would add support to the diagnosis of migraine.

Recommended action

- Check for an infective basis for the headache
- Carry out sinus X-rays if there is focal sinus tenderness or purulent nasal discharge
- Refer immediately to an accident and emergency department if there are any signs of meningeal irritation
- Administer IV benzylpenicillin prior to hospital transfer if there is a suspicion of meningococcal meningitis

Acute, recurrent headache

For most patients with acute, recurrent headache the diagnosis will be migraine or cluster headache (the former being commoner). Establishing a history of identical previous attacks (including, sometimes, focal neurological symptoms or signs) immediately lessens any anxiety regarding underlying structural brain disease.

Recommended action

- Any focal signs demand immediate referral
- Search hard for a history of previous similar attacks

Subacute, continuing headache

This clinical scenario, particularly in older people, raises the possibility of a structural process such as:

- brain tumour or abscess;

- subdural haematoma;

- cranial arteritis.

If cranial arteritis is suspected, an urgent erythrocyte sedimentation rate (ESR) or plasma viscosity should be arranged. If either is elevated, corticosteroids should be started immediately and the patient should be urgently referred.

For patients with space-occupying lesions, there will almost inevitably be other symptoms or focal neurological signs that suggest that possibility.

Recommended action

- Carry out an immediate ESR or plasma viscosity if there are any features of cranial arteritis
- If the headaches persist, consider early neurological referral

Chronic headache

Most patients seen in general practice (and outpatient departments) with chronic headache have tension headache. The history is usually one of months or years.

The relationship between cervical spondylosis and occipital headache is contentious. Finding radiological changes of spondylosis in, say, a man of 60 with chronic headache is insufficient to establish the spondylosis as the basis of the headache. Cervical spondylosis as a cause of occipital headache is likely only if the pain is associated with neck pain, and if there is limitation of, and pain during, neck movement.

In some patients, chronic pain in the region of the jaw or temple is related to temporomandibular joint dysfunction. For support, this diagnosis requires the presence of focal joint tenderness.

Recommended action

- If neck pathology seems the likely basis for an occipital headache, consider physiotherapy referral
- Try simple analgesics first if you suspect tension headache, but keep a check on the patient's analgesic intake
- If there is conspicuous temporomandibular joint tenderness, refer to a dental surgeon

Practice points

- The key to the accurate diagnosis of headache lies in the history, not the examination

- Careful enquiry (backed by accurate records) often establishes that a headache history is longer than the patient first implies

- A change in quality of an established headache syndrome or a newly evolving headache in an older person should prompt consideration of referral

- Most acute headache seen in general practice is due to non-specific infection. Both meningitis and subarachnoid haemorrhage are likely to be accompanied by signs of meningeal irritation. Tumour headache is almost inevitably accompanied by other neurological symptoms and sometimes by signs

Common fallacies

- That headache is a feature of chronic sinus disease, refractive errors or hypertension

- That chronic headache, without focal symptoms or signs, should raise a fear of structural disease

Dizziness

Epidemiology

Dizziness, or vertigo, figures substantially as a pre-eminent complaint in the workload of both general practitioners and neurologists. In Fry's experience, the symptoms accounted for 30 consultations per 2000 patients per annum.[2] In an outpatient neurology series, vertigo, dizziness or giddiness was a primary part of the patient's symptoms in 11 per cent of consultations.[9] A survey of patients in four general practices in London revealed that one in five responders had experienced dizziness within the previous month.[10] A more recent practice analysis concluded that 2.2 per cent of patients per year consulted regarding dizziness, amounting to 0.7 per cent of all consultations[11] (i.e. about half the figure in Fry's series).

Data on the underlying mechanism of dizziness, as seen by the general practitioner, are difficult to come by. Analysis by questionnaire is unable to provide diagnostic data, although one such analysis established that half of the patients with dizziness reported anxiety or agorophobic behaviour.[12] In a neurological outpatient setting, a breakdown of diagnosis in patients in whom vertigo, dizziness or giddiness was a primary complaint (though not necessarily the sole complaint) indicated that approximately half of the patients either had a psychiatric disorder or were not specifically diagnosed (Table 7).

When a patient presents to a general practitioner (or a neurologist) with vertigo or dizziness as the sole complaint, the likely diagnosis lies between:

- a psychiatric condition;

- an acute vestibular upset;

Underlying condition	Number
Primary psychiatric disorder*	109
Unknown	96
Acute or recurrent vestibulopathy	69
Syncope†	37
Epilepsy	36
Post-traumatic	31
Cerebrovascular disease	30
Benign positional vertigo	22
Multiple sclerosis	8
Meniérè's disease	2
Malignant intracranial tumour	2
Acoustic neuroma	1
Bell's palsy	1

*Hyperventilation (43), Conversion hysteria (32), Depression (23), Anxiety State (11).
†Includes vasovagal attacks, micturition and cough syncope
Adapted from Perkin.[9]

Table 7
Vertigo, dizziness and giddiness – underlying condition in a survey of 444 patients

- benign positional vertigo;

- a condition of unknown origin.

How can enquiry (and examination) help that diagnosis?

Important features in the history

The nature of the symptoms

- First, determine whether the patient has true vertigo (i.e. that there is an experience of rotation of the self or of the environment) or not.

- If so, does the vertigo occur in certain circumstances (e.g. while the patient is lying in bed at night), or is it random?

- Is there a history of similar attacks, perhaps months or years previously?

Accompanying symptoms

- In attacks of vertigo, the patient is necessarily ataxic.

- When a patient refers to ataxia accompanying the dizziness, determine whether there is objective evidence (i.e. from eyewitnesses) to support that contention.

- Is the symptom accompanied by tinnitus or deafness (suggesting an otological cause)?

- Is the symptom accompanied by palpitations, tingling and feelings of anxiety (suggesting acute panic attacks)?

Environmental factors

- Attacks of anxiety tend to occur in crowded places (supermarkets are the prime example), when driving or during stressful encounters.

- Attacks of benign positional vertigo are almost always noted when the patient lies down in bed, but specifically when the patient turns to one side.

Physical findings

Objective evidence of ataxia is usually missing in patients with non-specific dizziness, even if subjective unsteadiness has formed part of the history. In an acute vestibular insult, say of the right labyrinth, the patient has vertigo towards the left, tends to fall to the right on Romberg testing and has a nystagmus with the fast phase to the left.

Clinical scenarios

Conditions to consider in a patient with dizziness or vertigo are listed in Table 8.

Acute vertigo

In general practice, the most likely causes are an acute vestibular insult (vestibular neuronitis, labyrinthitis) or benign positional vertigo.

In an acute vestibular insult, there may be a history of prior upper respiratory tract infection and similar episodes in

Acute vestibulopathy (labyrinthitis, vestibular neuronitis)
Benign positional vertigo
Psychological mechanisms
Meniérè's disease
Cerebrovascular disease (rarely)
Epilepsy (rarely)
Acoustic neuroma (rarely)

Table 8
Conditions to consider as causes of dizziness or vertigo

family members. The vertigo is accompanied by vomiting and unsteadiness. The symptoms gradually resolve but the aftermath may be protracted in the elderly.

Benign positional vertigo produces characteristic attacks with head movement; attacks may be triggered by head positioning (Figure 2). A specific manoeuvre can then lead to the prevention of further attacks.

Treatment of vertigo has significant limitations. Several drugs have some vestibular sedative activity. The main choices are prochlorperazine, betahistine and cinnarizine. None of these drugs should be given on a long-term basis.

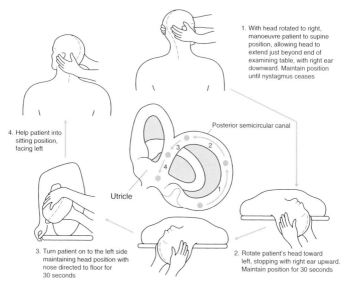

1. With head rotated to right, manoeuvre patient to supine position, allowing head to extend just beyond end of examining table, with right ear downward. Maintain position until nystagmus ceases

Posterior semicircular canal

4. Help patient into sitting position, facing left

Utricle

3. Turn patient on to the left side maintaining head position with nose directed to floor for 30 seconds

2. Rotate patient's head toward left, stopping with right ear upward. Maintain position for 30 seconds

Figure 2
Manoeuvre to relieve benign positional vertigo of right ear. (Directions of rotation should be reversed for the left ear.) Numbers in the labyrinth (centre) show position of debris as it moves around the posterior semicircular canal and into the utricle during the corresponding steps of the manoeuvre. Repeat the manoeuvre until nystagmus cannot be elicited
Adapted from Foster and Baloh,[13] with kind permission of WB Saunders Company.

Recommended action

- Carry out head positioning if you suspect benign positional vertigo. The positioning must result in nystagmus, not just vertigo, if you are confidently to make the diagnosis of benign positional vertigo

- Short-term vestibular sedatives are appropriate if you suspect a diagnosis of acute labyrinthitis or vestibular neuronitis

Recurrent episodic vertigo

Many patients with benign positional vertigo give a history of similar attacks in the past. In general practice, a common cause of recurrent attacks of vertigo is Meniérè's disease. Meniérè's disease is characterized by recurrent attacks of vertigo coupled with tinnitus and hearing loss, which eventually becomes permanent. Vestibular sedatives are the stand-by for acute attacks. Surgical intervention is sometimes needed if the attacks become intractable.

Recurrent vertigo can sometimes occur as a manifestation of either epilepsy or cerebrovascular disease. Neither is a sensible diagnostic option unless there are additional symptoms in the attacks to point to one or the other.

Recommended action

- If the history suggests previous attacks of benign positional vertigo treat as appropriate (see above)

- If there are accompanying features suggestive of Meniérè's disease, use vestibular sedatives for the acute attack

- If there are accompanying symptoms or unusual features in the attacks, consider neurological referral

Chronic vertigo, dizziness or dysequilibrium

The main organic basis for this problem is bilateral vestibular damage caused by streptomycin or gentamicin. The diagnosis is usually evident from the history of drug exposure. Many patients who have had an acute vestibular insult develop a chronic state of dizziness and a lack of confidence in walking. Typically they express fears of walking out of doors unless accompanied. There is some evidence that early referral for vestibular rehabilitation or balance retraining can be fruitful in lessening the duration and severity of the patient's symptoms.

Recommended action

- Early referral for vestibular rehabilitation is appropriate for any dizzy patient if the symptoms appear to be becoming chronic

Practice points

- Acute vertigo is most likely to be due to an acute vestibular insult or benign positional vertigo (when the cause can be identified)
- When acute attacks of dizziness are described in the absence of vertigo, psychological factors should be sought for
- Rather than prescribing long-term vestibular sedatives, referral for vestibular rehabilitation should be considered unless an acute bout of vertigo or dizziness settles rapidly

Common fallacies

- That bouts of vertigo triggered by neck rotation are due to vertebrobasilar insufficiency
- That chronic feelings of dysequilibrium or dizziness, in the absence of neurological signs, are likely to be due to central nervous system disease

Altered consciousness and delirium

Epidemiology

Fry calculated that epilepsy and syncope accounted for 20 consultations per 2000 patients per annum.[2] In a recently published community-based study,[3] the age- and sex-adjusted incidence rate for epilepsy (including single seizures) was 57 per 100,000, which is very close to the figure that Fry quoted (1–2 per 2000) for annual incidence. In outpatient neurological practice, epilepsy (including single seizures) and syncopal attacks account for 12.5 per cent of all consultations.[4] There are no data indicating how often delirium (assuming one can agree on the criteria for its diagnosis) is encountered in general practice, although it is suggested that 10–25 per cent of patients aged over 65 years admitted to general medical units suffer from 'confusion'.[14]

ALTERED CONSCIOUSNESS

Eyewitness accounts are crucial to the better understanding of the cause of loss of consciousness. Many mistakes in interpretation can be avoided by eliminating the use of ambiguous terminology. What does the patient mean by a blackout? When observers insist that consciousness was not lost in an attack, is that simply because the eyes were still open?

Important features in the history

Prodromal symptoms

Patients who faint do not lose consciousness abruptly. They have warning symptoms in terms of light-headedness, fading of vision or hearing, sweating and a sense of the likelihood of losing consciousness. Auras before attacks of epilepsy are important since they indicate a focal origin for the seizure. Such auras are very brief and often difficult for the patient to discuss. Patients whose syncope is due to a cardiac arrhythmia may well notice chest pain or palpitations before loss of consciousness.

Features of the attack

The overlap of the clinical features of syncope and epilepsy is greater than has been previously realized. During syncopal attacks, many patients may vocalize and show limb movements (though never the tonic–clonic progression of a generalized seizure). A bitten tongue almost inevitably indicates an epileptic event. The fall during syncope is much less abrupt than in an epileptic event.

The setting of an attack

Certain types of syncope occur in particular settings.

- Micturition syncope mainly affects males (not necessarily older men) and leads to syncope during micturition, almost always in the night and usually after alcohol ingestion

- Cough syncope is triggered by paroxysmal coughing, usually in a person with chronic obstructive airways disease

- Vasovagal syncope tends to occur in the upright position (occasionally while sitting) and is triggered by an emotional upset, prolonged standing or the experience of a painful procedure.

The aftermath of the attack

Patients who faint usually recover rapidly, although they may faint again if they return too rapidly to the upright position.

Drop attacks tend to occur in older women without warning, and the patient falls forward. Patients may attempt to save themselves and recall the pavement coming to meet them. They can usually return quickly to the upright position, unless injured, although their confidence is often shaken.

After an epileptic event, particularly of the tonic–clonic type, the patient is drowsy; indeed, the patient may sleep deeply for several hours.

Clinical scenarios

Apparent syncopal attack

Recommended action

- If the attack is vasovagal in type, further action is unnecessary in a younger person

- Episodes in older people, while still sometimes vasovagal in nature, are more likely to represent a cardiac dysrhythmia or postural hypotension. Check the patient's standing and lying blood pressure, assess the cardiac status and arrange an electrocardiogram. Consider referral

- If the history is typical for cough or micturition syncope, advise the patient about avoidance measures

Apparent seizure

Recommended action

- All patients suspected of having had a seizure should be referred for specialist opinion

- It is probably unreasonable to initiate treatment for a single seizure

- Patients who have had an episode of unexpected loss of consciousness should be advised not to drive

DELIRIUM

Delirium is defined as a fluctuating disturbance of consciousness with reduced awareness of the environment that has developed relatively acutely. Additional features are impaired attention and altered cognition.[15] The problem is triggered by a variety of medical illnesses, intoxications, withdrawal states or metabolic disorders. The terms 'delirium' and 'confusion' tend to be used interchangeably to describe the same clinical state. Patients in this situation often show an altered sleep cycle, with the confusion or agitation becoming more apparent at night. Delirium, or an acute confusional state, is relatively uncommon in the young, and is usually then attributable to drug intoxication. The problem is more complex in the elderly. In both groups, however, a systematic approach to assessment is needed if the underlying aetiology is to be discovered.

Important features in the history

Predisposing illnesses

Many intercurrent illnesses can trigger a confusional state in the elderly, particularly if there is already some degree of cognitive impairment. A careful search needs to be made for evidence of a renal tract or respiratory infection. A mild stroke, or a silent myocardial infarct, may have a similar effect. Evidence of recent-onset diabetes should be sought.

Drug intake

The elderly are particularly prone to the adverse effects of certain drugs that are tolerated without difficulty by younger people. Benzhexol, for example, if started in incautious doses (e.g. 6 mg daily) provokes confusion in about one-third of elderly patients. A careful drug history therefore is mandatory. Alcohol intake may be relevant, and information from carers or relatives is important in this context.

Management issues

The confused patient is likely to return sooner to his or her normal cognitive state at home than in hospital. This ideal can be realized only if the patient does not have a serious underlying illness and only if the patient's relatives are able to cope with the situation.

Recommended action

- Identification and treatment of the underlying precipitant is essential

- Repeated attempts should be made by the carers to reorientate the patient

- Sedation is best avoided. If it is absolutely necessary use intramuscular haloperidol (0.5–10 mg). Alternatively, low oral doses (1–10 mg/day) can be used

Practice points

- Many syncopal events do not require specialist opinion
- Suspect a cardiac basis for funny turns in the elderly
- Always remember to check standing and lying blood pressure in older patients who complain of faint-like feelings
- Refer any patient whom you suspect has had a seizure
- Search hard for a trigger in the patient with delirium
- Use sedation sparingly in the confused patient

Common fallacies

- That any limb movement during a 'faint-like' episode suggests epilepsy
- That minor epileptic events do not require the patient to stop driving
- That heavy sedation is the norm in the management of the confused patient

Epidemiology

There are no data from general practice indicating how frequently patients present with weakness. In neurological outpatient practice, weakness figures as a feature among the complaints of the 26.5 per cent of patients who do not have a specific diagnosis, and accounts for about 5 per cent of that total.[4] Usually, however, the basis of a complaint of weakness is discovered.

Important features in the history

What is meant by weakness?

Many patients confuse weakness with inco-ordination, bradykinesia or even loss of sensation. Establish exactly what they mean if they describe weakness.

Distribution

Unilateral weakness is likely to be due either to a disturbance of the spinal cord or of brain function. Establish if the arm and leg are equally affected.

Focal weakness of an arm or leg may still reflect central nervous system disease, but introduces the possibility of a disturbance of a nerve root or peripheral nerve.

Weakness of all four limbs may be brain stem, spinal cord or peripheral in origin, the last either due to muscle or peripheral nerve dysfunction.

Distribution within the limb is important. Peripheral neuropathies tend to cause distal weakness whereas primary muscle diseases tend to cause proximal weakness.

Mode of onset

Most strokes present acutely or subacutely. Spinal cord compression from a metastasis develops rapidly, whereas spinal cord compression from spondylitic disease or a benign tumour develops more gradually. Primary muscle disease (e.g. polymyositis) can present acutely or chronically.

Accompanying symptoms

Although disruption of spinal cord, nerve root or peripheral nerve function should lead to both motor and sensory symptoms (and signs), motor manifestations may predominate. Pure motor symptoms are obligatory if the problem is in the anterior horn cell (motor neurone disease), the neuromuscular junction (myasthenia gravis) or the muscle itself (the myopathies, polymyositis).

The nature of the weakness

When the motor problem is in the brain or spinal cord (causing an upper motor neurone weakness) the patient sometimes describes the limb, or limbs, as being heavy or stiff. The patient may notice that the limb jerks repetitively in certain positions or that the leg (or legs) drag when walking. In multiple sclerosis, it is particularly characteristic for there to be a tendency for the legs to become 'heavy' as the patient walks for a critical distance. Muscle fatigue is suggestive of myasthenia gravis, although a complaint of global fatigue is of no value in differential diagnosis.

Clinical scenarios

The weak hand

First, establish what the patient means by 'weakness'. If the patient describe clumsiness or a paucity of movement, remember to look for bradykinesia if muscle strength is intact. Check this by asking the patient to polish the back of one hand with the other, or sequentially touch each finger with the thumb. In early Parkinsonism, the movement gradually slows in speed and reduces in amplitude. The same phenomena can be recorded by asking for a specimen of the patient's handwriting.

If the hand is weak, attempt to assess whether the weakness is confined to muscles supplied by a particular nerve or whether all the hand muscles are affected. Are there lower motor neurone features, such as wasting or fasciculation? The common entrapment neuropathies of the upper limb affect the median and ulnar nerves. Median nerve entrapment sometimes presents with motor deficit; ulnar nerve entrapment very commonly does. If the patient has problems with a specific task, watch the patient perform it. In writer's cramp (one of the focal dystonias), the hand is strong but the patient uses excessive force when writing, with altered grip resulting in distorted script.

Weak legs

The problem may be symmetrical or asymmetrical; if asymmetrical, the patient may be unaware of the involvement of the less affected limb.

Predominant distal weakness (with the feet tending to flop) suggests a peripheral neuropathy.

Predominant proximal weakness (difficulty in climbing or descending stairs, difficulty getting out of a chair) suggests a primary muscle problem.

When spinal cord disease causes weakness, particularly with multiple sclerosis, the patient may notice excessive muscle fatigue, with increasing weakness and stiffness as walking continues.

The floppy foot

Unilateral foot drop is usually peripheral in origin and is usually the manifestation of a lateral popliteal (common peroneal) palsy or of a lesion of the fourth lumbar nerve root (Figure 3). Both may eventually be accompanied by wasting of the anterior tibial compartment. The patient lifts the leg excessively at the hip to overcome the problem.

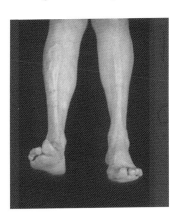

Figure 3
Left foot drop in a patient with a lateral popliteal palsy

Rarely, foot drop is due to a brain lesion. In this case, the muscle is stiff and the patient is more likely to drag the foot when walking, causing differential shoe wear.

Practice points

- A presenting complaint of weakness is likely to merit neurological referral, since the vast majority of patients with this problem require further investigation, either by electromyography or neuroimaging

- If there is no weakness but the patient complains of problems with a specific task (e.g. writing) observe the patient while he or she carries out that task

- If weakness is not confirmed but the patient complains of paucity of movement, check for bradykinesia and consider a diagnosis of early Parkinson's disease

- Mastering the examination of representative muscles supplied by the median and ulnar nerves in the hand will aid diagnosis of the common entrapment neuropathies of the upper limb

Common fallacies

- That a feeling of global weakness or fatigue is likely to be neurological

- That a complaint of weakness excludes malfunction of the extrapyramidal system (Parkinson's disease) or of the cerebellum

- That a complaint of weakness alone excludes disorders in which sensory function could also be affected

Numbness and paraesthesiae

As with muscle weakness, there are no data from general practice studies as to the frequency with which patients present with either numbness or paraesthesiae. Both of these symptoms are often more nebulous complaints than weakness, with a correspondingly higher representation among the undiagnosed patients (30 per cent of that total if limb pain is included).

Inportant features in the history

What is meant by numbness or paraesthesiae?

Ask the patient whether the numbness is subjective or whether there is objective loss to self-testing.

Patients with spinothalamic loss will notice loss of temperature awareness in the affected part (e.g. when taking a bath).

Patients with posterior column loss in the hand may complain of clumsiness or difficulty in identifying or manipulating objects if the object cannot be seen. Another symptom of posterior column loss is a feeling of tightness, as if a bandage is tied around the limb or the trunk.

Patients describe paraesthesiae in different ways. Recording their own description is appropriate.

Distribution

Patients with peripheral neuropathy complain of peripheral sensory symptoms, typically beginning in the feet and later in the hands. Peripheral sensory symptoms are very rarely due to limb vascular disease unless an individual digital nerve is ischaemic. A sensory problem that ascends on to the trunk cannot be due to a peripheral cause and must represent a spinal cord lesion (Figure 4). Patients with a

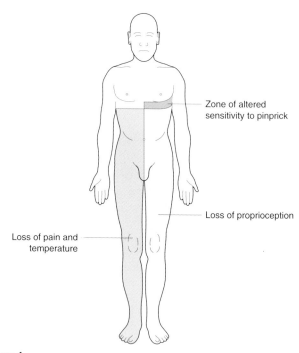

Zone of altered sensitivity to pinprick

Loss of proprioception

Loss of pain and temperature

Figure 4
A left sided spinal cord lesion (Brown–Séquard lesion). There is altered joint position sense in the left leg, but altered pain and temperature sensitivity in the right leg

peripheral nerve disorder may deny sensory symptoms, or those symptoms may occupy only part of the distribution of the particular nerve. On the other hand, patients with carpal tunnel syndrome may complain that the limb pain or tingling extends substantially beyond median nerve territory. For many patients with sensory symptoms the problem is rather nebulous, and it proves difficult to pinpoint the patient to a particular distribution in the limb.

Triggering factors

Certain features of the patient's history can strongly suggest either the exact site of origin of the sensory symptoms or their underlying cause.

Nocturnal pain and paraesthesiae are almost pathognomonic of carpal tunnel syndrome. The patient wakes with a numb or tingling hand (or hands) which they shake until the sensation subsides. The symptoms are much less prominent during the day.

Electric-shock sensations which radiate down the spine or into the limbs during neck flexion are known as Lhermitte's phenomenon. They are associated with pathology in the posterior columns of the cervical spinal cord and, in younger people, are typically a manifestation of multiple sclerosis.

Clinical scenarios

Numb feet

The commonest cause of gradually evolving numbness or tingling in the feet (typically commencing in the toes) is a peripheral neuropathy. The commonest cause of this, outside tropical countries, is diabetes. Supportive evidence for a diagnosis of peripheral neuropathy comes from finding absent ankle jerks and distal sensory loss, either cutaneous (light touch and pinprick) or posterior column (vibration sense and joint-position sense).

The risk of developing a symptomatic neuropathy in a previously unaffected diabetic patient rises to at least 15 per cent by 25 years of the illness, though a far higher percentage will have objective evidence of neurological dysfunction. The most common neuropathy is a distal symmetrical form with predominant sensory involvement and origin in the lower limbs. Involvement of autonomic fibres produces postural hypotension, loss of sweating and sphincter disturbances. In some patients, according to the type of nerve fibre affected, the symptoms include burning limb sensations of considerable severity.

Although there are treatment interventions which may alleviate some of the symptoms (amitriptyline, carbamazepine and gabapentin have been used for that purpose) critical diabetic control is mandatory. Intensive diabetic control significantly reduces the risk of developing neuropathy.

One numb foot

Although a peripheral neuropathy can be asymmetrical, numbness confined to one foot is likely to be due to peripheral nerve or nerve root dysfunction. If the patient has a lateral popliteal palsy, the dorsiflexors of the foot will be weak, plantar flexion will be normal, and the ankle jerk intact. If there is involvement of the fifth lumbar nerve root, the medial aspect of the foot may be numb; if there is involvement of the first sacral nerve root, the lateral aspect of the foot may be numb. With the latter, the ankle jerk is likely to be absent or depressed; with the former it will be normal.

Numb hands

Numb hands may be the result of bilateral carpal tunnel syndrome. The symptoms are often diffusely distributed and typically nocturnal. Alternatively, it may be that the patient has a cervical cord lesion. Multiple sclerosis would be a likely cause in a younger person, but perhaps more likely in an older person would be either cervical myelopathy due to disc degeneration or a peripheral neuropathy presenting in the upper limbs – an unusual occurrence. The presence of a Lhermitte phenomenon in a younger patient would favour a diagnosis of multiple sclerosis. Reflex changes associated with cervical spondylosis include a depressed or absent triceps reflex (compression of the seventh cervical nerve root or, sometimes, the sixth cervical nerve root) and depression or absence of the biceps and supinator reflexes (compression of the fifth cervical nerve root or, sometimes, the sixth cervical nerve root).

One numb hand

The most common cause of numbness isolated to a part of one hand are nerve root entrapment (fifth, sixth or seventh cervical) or a nerve entrapment syndrome (e.g. carpal tunnel syndrome or an ulnar nerve lesion).

A cervical root problem that produces hand numbness or paraesthesiae is likely to be accompanied by limb or neck pain and possibly reflex changes. Finding degenerative changes in the cervical spine on X-ray is not sufficient to establish the changes as the basis for the patient's symptoms. Degenerative changes in the neck in older patients are the norm.

Carpal tunnel syndrome is likely to be suggested by a particular pattern of nocturnal symptoms. Many ulnar nerve lesions are relatively asymptomatic. If sensory symptoms and signs occur (and they may not) the patient is likely to complain of altered sensation along the ulnar border of the hand, extending into the little finger. Often the sensory changes do not extend to the limit of the cutaneous distribution of the nerve. Sometimes there are bilateral findings despite the symptoms being unilateral.

Practice points

- Nocturnal tingling, numbness or pain in the hand is likely to be due to a carpal tunnel syndrome

- Isolated limb numbness or paraesthesiae is a recognized, though uncommon, presentation of nerve root compression

- Patients with a suspected peripheral neuropathy are likely to have depressed or absent ankle jerks

Common fallacies

- That any young person with numbness or paraesthesiae inevitably has multiple sclerosis

- That sensory symptoms or signs in mononeuropathies (lesions of individual peripheral nerves) will match the full extent of the distribution of the affected nerve

Stroke

Epidemiology

Fry estimated an annual incidence rate for stroke of 15–20 per 10,000 population, with an annual consulting rate, for the same population, of 75–100 cases.[2] In the recently published UK Survey of General Practice, the age- and sex-adjusted rate for a first cerebrovascular event was 205 per 100,000 of the population.[3] It has been estimated that over 80 per cent of stroke survivors are living in the community 1 year after their stroke; of these, at least 25 per cent are wholly dependent upon their immediate carer and a further 30 per cent require regular support (Table 9).[16]

Impending stroke

Many completed strokes, particularly those due to cerebral infarction, are preceded by one or more transient episodes

80%	Infarction
10%	Intracerebral haemorrhage
5%	Subarachnoid haemorrhage
5%	Uncertain

Table 9
Distribution of stroke type

of altered neurological function, usually lasting minutes but, by definition, for anything up to 24 hours. These episodes are transient ischaemic attacks (TIAs). Put the other way, TIAs are followed by a completed stroke in about 35 per cent of cases over a 5-year period. Antiplatelet agents, typically aspirin, or an aspirin–dipyridamole mixture, reduce that stroke risk by about 20 per cent. When the transient ischaemic attack has been triggered by a carotid stenosis of more than 70 per cent (more especially 80 per cent), surgical intervention (endarterectomy) significantly lessens risk for stroke, compared with medical treatment, over the subsequent 3 years. Patients in atrial fibrillation of non-rheumatic origin have a substantially higher risk of ischaemic stroke than patients who are in sinus rhythm.

Episodes suggestive of TIA include:

- transient altered speech;

- loss of vision confined to one eye;

- temporary altered function of an arm and leg on the same side of the body, whether as weakness, numbness or clumsiness.

It is unreasonable to assume attacks of vertigo or dizziness are due to ischaemia unless there are suggestive accompanying symptoms. Brief episodes of scintillations or flashing lights in older people may be ischaemic in origin, but they may also be migrainous.

Stroke in younger individuals

Certain possibilities need to be considered with TIAs or strokes occur in a younger individual.

Carotid or vertebral dissection

Dissection of the carotid or vertebral arteries as a cause of stroke is more common than was previously recognised.

Some of the patients will have had recent neck trauma or manipulation. Headache is a prominent component, often centred above the eye in carotid dissection and in the region of the mastoid in vertebral dissection. A Horner's syndrome occurs in about 50 per cent of cases of carotid dissection. A high index of suspicion is needed.

Cardiac embolization

In younger people with stroke, embolization from the heart is a strong possiblity. There may not be a cardiac history. Careful examination of the heart is essential.

Cerebral venous thrombosis

Modern imaging techniques have established that this is a not uncommon cause of stroke. It may present with features suggesting raised intracranial pressure or with a stroke-like event. There should be particular suspicion regarding the diagnosis in young women on the pill, and in women who are pregnant or who have recently delivered.

Recommended action

- With a suggestive history, check the blood pressure, the heart rhythm and the carotid pulses

- All patients with a TIA or minor stroke require urgent hospital appraisal. It is probably reasonable to start such patients (at least those with TIA) on aspirin (75 mg daily) pending the hospital appointment

- TIAs that persist despite aspirin therapy require hospital reappraisal

---

Situations that mimic stroke or TIA

Transient hypoglycaemia

A prominent feature of a hypoglycaemic attack in a diabetic subject can be focal neurological deficit (e.g. a hemiplegia).

When supposed TIAs are occurring in a diabetic subject, check the diabetic control.

Transient global amnesia

Typically an episode of transient global amnesia lasts for several hours. Patients fail to register ongoing memory, although they often function reasonably well in everyday tasks. They subsequently fail to recall events during this period. Transient global amnesia usually occurs in single episodes and is benign.

Migraine

In the early stages of migraine, attacks of focal neurological dysfunction can occur without headache (aura). The dysfunction may include altered vision in a homonymous distribution or altered limb function. Suggestions as to the correct diagnosis would be the age of the patient (typically young) and a family history of migraine. Nevertheless, referral is advisable.

The established stroke

Most stroke patients at home have care from a relative. Up to 14 per cent of such carers give up their own employment to fulfil their responsibility.[17] General practitioners represent the most common point of contact for stroke patients.[18] Issues that require ongoing appraisal in the stroke patient include:

- hypertension control;

- the need for community services;

- the recognition of concomitant problems, including depression.

Depression is estimated to occur in some 15 per cent of stroke patients who are in the home environment.[19]

Depression needs to be distinguished from emotional lability, a common problem in patients who have had bilateral hemisphere strokes. Depressive illness in the stroke patient is likely to respond to conventional antidepressant therapy.

Depression may well develop in the carer, particularly if over-optimistic accounts of recovery potential are given.[20] Appropriate support for the carer is critical. Periodic respite care can give the carer much needed rest from the continuing commitment, as can attendance of the stroke patient at day centres where psychological support, allied with physical therapy for the patient, can be offered.

Recommended action

- Regular review of the physical and emotional needs of the stroke patient at home is essential for the welfare both of the patient and the carer. Early recognition of depressive symptoms, either in the patient or the carer, is to be encouraged; such symptoms require vigorous intervention

Practice points

- Recognition of TIAs requires early hospital referral
- Aspirin is of value in reducing stroke risk in TIA patients. Recent evidence suggests concomitant hypertension must be controlled if aspirin is used

Common fallacies

- That episodes of dizziness and vertigo in older subjects triggered by neck rotation can be attributed to vertebrobasilar insufficiency
- That loss of consciousness is a feature of hemisphere TIAs

Migraine and tension headache

Data on the prevalance of migraine and tension headache have already been given.

MIGRAINE

Migraine affects about 12–15 per cent of the UK population

- Women are three times more affected than men
- Attacks are typically recurrent
- Severity is very variable
- Bilateral attacks are just as likely as unilateral attacks, and throbbing pain is by no means inevitable (Figure 5). Attacks are not likely to continue for more than 3 days
- When migraine attacks are said to be occurring at weekly intervals or more frequently, psychological factors are likely to be contributing
- Migraine with aura (e.g. visual scintillations) is far less common than migraine without aura

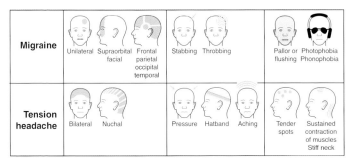

| | Unilateral | Supraorbital facial | Frontal parietal occipital temporal | Stabbing | Throbbing | Pallor or flushing | Photophobia Phonophobia |
| Migraine | | | | | | | |

| | Bilateral | Nuchal | Pressure | Hatband | Aching | Tender spots | Sustained contraction of muscles Stiff neck |
| Tension headache | | | | | | | |

Figure 5
Some of the clinical characteristics of migraine and tension headache

Specific issues

Management of attacks

Simple analgesics suffice for many patients. For some patients addition of metoclopramide to paracetemol enhances absorption of the latter drug and improves benefit. Codeine derivatives are best avoided. If simple analgesics fail, or are vomited, a non-steroidal in the form of a suppository can be used, supported, if necessary, by domperidone suppositories (30 mg).[21] If the patient is ill at home and unable to tolerate or contemplate a suppository, consider intramuscular diclofenac (75 mg) with intramuscular chlorpromazine (25–50 mg).

When these measures regularly fail, the general practitioner can try a triptan derivative. There are several choices.

Prevention of attacks

Patients should be advised not to miss meals and to avoid sleeping in. Certain foods (e.g. cheese, chocolate, citrus fruit, Bovril or Marmite) may trigger attacks, but this is a factor in no more than 10% of the migraine population. Alcohol (particularly red wine) is a potent trigger in some patients.

Prophylaxis

When migraine attacks are occurring frequently and are poorly controlled by medication, prophylactic therapy is worth considering. The usual causes of failure of action of a prophylactic agent are poor compliance, inadequate dosage or insufficient duration of treatment. Generally, a prophylactic drug is given for about 6 months and then withdrawn (sometimes gradually) to assess ongoing need. Drugs to consider initially are the beta-blockers, sodium valproate, pizotifen and amitriptyline (Table 9). Other

Drug	Dose range	Disadvantages
Atenolol	25–100 mg/day	Contraindicated if patient has asthma, heart failure or peripheral vascular disease
Propranolol LA	80–320 mg/day	Contraindicated if patient has asthma, heart failure or peripheral vascular disease
Metoprolol	100–200 mg/day	Contraindicated if patient has asthma or peripheral vascular disease
Sodium valproate	600–1500 mg/day	Teratogenic Weight gain
Pizotifen	1.5–3.0 mg/day	Sedation Weight gain
Amitriptyline	10–75 mg/day	Sedation Anticholinergic effects

Table 9
Prophylactic agents in migraine

agents for prophylaxis are best used in association with hospital input.

Migraine and the contraceptive pill

In some patients, migraine worsens with the combined oral contraceptive (COC). If a patient on the COC shows a change in migraine pattern (particularly a switch from migraine without aura to migraine with aura) then the COC should be stopped immediately.

Relative contraindications to COC use include:

- migraine with aura;

- migraine without aura in the presence of other stroke risk factors;

- use of ergot derivatives for attacks.

Migraine and pregnancy

Migraine tends to improve in pregnancy. If prophylaxis is thought essential, propranolol is the drug of choice. The drug can be continued during lactation.

Migraine and hormone replacement therapy

Hormone replacement therapy can be given to patients with migraine.

A sudden change in migraine

A sudden increase in the frequency of migraine or a change from migraine without aura to migraine with aura may be a reflection of non-compliance with prophylactic therapy. Nevertheless, such a change should prompt hospital referral.

Very frequent migraine

Very frequent migraine attacks are often a reflection of underlying psychological factors or may be due to the concurrence of migraine with tension headache. If the latter, amitriptyline is the drug of choice for prophylaxis. In some patients, the problem is one of medication-misuse headache.

TENSION HEADACHE

Tension headache, or tension-type headache, is more easily described than defined. It may occur episodically or as a chronic daily headache. Typically the pain is generalized (although it can be unilateral). It is less severe than migraine (Table 10) and is described as band-like, vice-like, sharp or stabbing. It may be accompanied by nausea,

	Migraine	Tension headache
Distribution	Often unilateral	Seldom unilateral
Character	Pulsatile, throbbing, intense	Band-like, tight, aching
Frequency	Not more than weekly	Often daily
Duration	Maximum 72 hours	May be continuous
Nausea	Almost always	Seldom
Vomiting	Perhaps 50%	Virtually never
Focal neurological symptoms	In patients with aura (perhaps 15% of all patients)	Never
Photophobia and phonophobia	Commonplace	Rare

Table 10
Differentiation of tension headache from migraine

but not by vomiting (see Figure 5). In some patients a depressive illness underlies the headache. More posteriorly placed tension headaches may arise from derangement of the cervical spine, although the association is over-estimated.

Some patients with very frequent tension-type headache have medication misuse headache. The association is best described with ergotamine, but it has now also been encountered with patients abusing the triptan drugs. Other drugs that can cause this syndrome include aspirin, codeine combinations and non-steroidal anti-inflammatory agents. If there is suspicion of analgesic abuse the offending agent must be withdrawn. Even then, it may take months for improvement to occur.

Specific issues

Management

If the tension-type headache is episodic, simple analgesia is appropriate. Codeine derivatives should be avoided. Analysis of depressive symptoms is worthwhile. Physiotherapy in the form of massage, mobilization or manipulation may be beneficial if a cervical basis for the problem appears likely.

Chronic tension-type headaches are much more difficult to manage. Amitriptyline is the drug of choice, in doses up to about 75 mg daily, but intolerance is common. Many patients fail to respond and seek solutions through alternative medicine, including acupuncture, homeopathy and aromatherapy.

When to refer

Many patients with chronic tension headaches believe that their problem is due to brain disease, and in particular a brain tumour. They may insist on a neurological referral. If that request is granted it should be after the above therapeutic measures have been attempted. Patients should be told that they are being referred for a consultant opinion, not simply to have a scan performed which would in fact be irrelevant to their needs.

Practice points

- Most patients with migraine and tension headache can be managed in general practice
- Reasons for referral include a changing pattern of headache, resistance to drug therapy and the patient's fear of more serious underlying pathology

Common fallacies

- That chronic sinus disease is a cause of headache
- That refractive errors are a common cause of tension-type headache
- That headaches related to disease of the ears, teeth or temporomandibular joints can occur without symptoms referrable to those structures

Multiple sclerosis

Epidemiology

An approximate figure for the prevalance of multiple sclerosis (MS) in the UK is 100 per 100,000. A community-based prevalance study reported an incidence rate of 7 per 100,000 per year.[3] Fry estimated that 10 consultations per year would occur in a general practice of 10,000 patients.[2] In neurology outpatients, the condition accounts for 3.5 per cent of consultations.[4] The condition pursues a remitting–relapsing course, at least initially, in about 80 per cent of patients, and a progressive course from the onset in about 15 per cent (primary progressive MS). After 8–10 years, the majority of remitting–relapsing cases enter a secondary progressive course (secondary progressive MS) (Figure 6). About 65 per cent of the patients are women. The peak age of onset is around 30 years. Onset is rare under the age of 15 and beyond the age of 60. About 50 per cent of MS patients are independent and still able to walk 15 years after the onset of the disease.

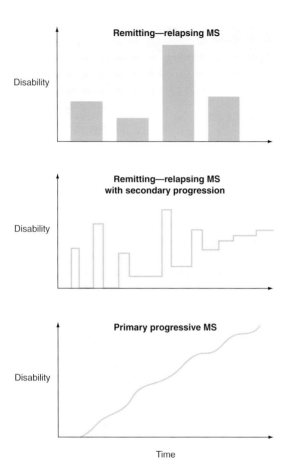

Figure 6
Disability with time in different types of MS

Specific issues

Early symptoms

The early symptoms of MS are often nebulous and difficult
to distinguish from the non-specific symptoms encountered

very frequently in outpatient practice. However, certain complaints should alert the general practitioner to the possibility of MS.

- Lhermitte's sign – patients describe electric shock sensations radiating down the spine during neck flexion. In young people the cause is almost always MS

- Heat or exercise-induced symptoms – many MS patients describe transient symptoms (e.g. clumsiness, heaviness of the legs or blurred vision), which appear while walking or taking a hot bath and which then resolve

- Unilateral vision loss – optic neuritis produces eye pain followed by blurring or loss of vision, usually confined to one eye. The fundus may appear normal, or the optic disc may be swollen. Typically there is a central scotoma (Figure 7)

Because of the difficulty in determining the importance of nebulous sensory or other symptoms, neurological referral is usually appropriate. If referral does not take place, a careful record of the episode should be made in case it has bearing on the diagnosis in the future.

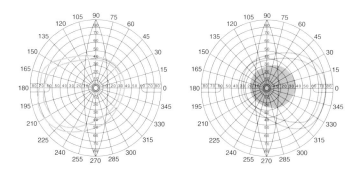

Figure 7
A large right central scotoma in a patient with optic neuritis

Acute exacerbations

Most MS patients, though not all, will be known to a neurology department. Individual consultants will vary as to whether they wish to be involved in decision-making about treatment of acute exacerbations. Many exacerbations do not receive treatment. Severe episodes require admission. For lesser episodes in which treatment is likely to be helpful (by shortening the duration of the event) it is probably reasonable to initiate therapy using oral prednisolone, say 60 mg daily for a week, then 30 mg daily for a week, and finally 15 mg daily for a week. If the response is unsatisfactory, the issue can be discussed with the relevant consultant.

Multiple sclerosis and pregnancy

Women can be advised that attacks will not increase during pregnancy, but that the relapse rate approximately doubles during the first 3 months after delivery. This does not, however, appear to influence the long-term course of the disease.

Multiple sclerosis and external events

Although individual patients report worsening of their condition after, say, a traumatic event, they can be advised that there is no evidence that operations, anaesthetics, dental extractions or vaccination procedures affect the course of the disease. Stress may temporarily exacerbate symptoms but it does not have a longer-lasting effect.

Beta-interferon

Assuming that beta-interferon continues to be funded, referral for consideration of its use should be confined to patients under the age of 50 who have remitting–relapsing disease and who are continuing to have relapses.

Established multiple sclerosis

All too easily, patients with established MS are lost sight of, both from the hospital service and from general practice. Substantial issues relating to the patient's care and welfare become correspondingly neglected. Ideally, the input of an MS specialist nurse, working in tandem with the hospital service and general practice, allows early identification of potential problems. Areas that should be covered include:

- bladder problems;

- depression;

- sexual disorders;

- physiotherapy;

- occupational therapy;

- respite care.

Bladder problems.

Bladder problems are common in established MS. Symptoms do not accurately reflect the state of bladder emptying. Drugs (e.g. oxybutynin and tolterodine), can ease urgency and frequency but may exacerbate a tendency to urinary retention. Bladder ultrasound studies before and after micturition are invaluable when planning treatment. Intermittent self-catheterization can be of major value in those patients who are retaining substantial volumes of urine (>100ml) after micturition. Even in the absence of overt urinary tract infection, periodic urine culture is advisable. Occult urinary tract infection is liable to aggravate spasticity.

Depression

Depression is far more common in MS patients than euphoria. Failure to recognize its presence is a far greater bar to its relief than resistance to therapy.

Sexual disorders

Impotence is common in the male MS patient and may well respond to sildenafil.

Physiotherapy

Periodic review of gait patterns by a physiotherapist is relevant for those patients with walking problems, as is regular appraisal of walking aids if they are in use.

Occupational therapy

As patients become more disabled, there is an increasing need to appraise their home environment. Through periodic home visits, the occupational therapist can assess the activities of daily living and make recommendations regarding bath aids, stair aids, special chairs and so on. If the local hospital has a multidisciplinary rehabilitation unit, periodic referrals can allow an efficient reappraisal of the patient's needs.

Respite care

As the burden of care increases, so does the physical and emotional stress on the carer. Regular periods of respite care, during which an active programme of rehabilitation can be pursued, produce ongoing benefit for both parties.

Practice points

- Certain complaints, including exercise- or heat-induced symptoms and tingling sensations in the spine on neck flexion, should alert the doctor to the possibility of MS

- Many MS relapses do not warrant corticosteroids. Of those that do, some can be managed by oral corticosteroids

- When disability is becoming more prominent, regular reviews of the patient's needs by paramedical staff are invaluable

Common fallacies

- That a single demyelinating event establishes a diagnosis of MS

- That patients with established MS will inevitably be known to the hospital service, obviating the need for general practice involvement

- That any fresh symptom in an MS patient, whatever its nature, can be attributed to MS

Epilepsy

Epidemiology

The age- and sex-adjusted rate for seizure disorders (including single fits) in the UK survey already referred to was 57 per 100,000.[3] In Fry's general practice data, epilepsy accounted for 60 consultations per year in a population of 10,000.[2] In neurological outpatient practice epilepsy (including single seizures) accounted for 10.4 per cent of referrals.[4] It has been calculated that a general practice with 10,000 patients will contain 50 patients who are on anticonvulsants.[22]

Patients with a diagnosis of epilepsy must have had at least two seizure events. A single seizure does not constitute epilepsy, since some patients never experience a recurrence.

Data suggest that over 90 per cent of patients with an epileptic event are referred to hospital,[23] but after an average of four visits patients are either discharged or fail to attend for further follow-up. The major burden of care, therefore, rests in general practice. Analysis of this process reveals problems in continuity of care, inappropriate drug therapy and poor general practitioner–patient communication, coupled with poor patient compliance with medication and low levels of patient knowledge.[24] When appraising the need for patient review, general practitioners themselves suggest that an appointment at 6-monthly intervals would be appropriate.[25]

Specific issues

The first seizure

A first seizure merits hospital referral. Increasingly all such patients are imaged and have electrophysiology performed. Eye witness accounts are invaluable in assessment and details should be included in the referral letter. Indeed, any eyewitness should be encouraged to accompany the patient to the appointment. Careful enquiry of the patient should be made in case there is a history of previous attacks in the past. The patient should be immediately told to stop driving and warned that if the diagnosis of a seizure is sustained, driving will not be allowed (in the UK) for 12 months. At present it is the usual practice not to treat a single seizure. Therefore, treatment should not be initiated before the first hospital appointment.

Established epilepsy

Patients with a history of two or more seizures have epilepsy. It is well worthwhile giving them the details of the British Epilepsy Association (Anstey House, Hanover Square, Leeds, LS19 7XY; Freephone helpline 0808-800/5050; e-mail helpline@bea.org.uk). A clear understanding should be reached between the general practitioner and the hospital service as to who is providing ongoing care. Nothing is to be served by two doctors separately adjusting medication. If the patient is solely under general practitioner care, 6-monthly reviews would seem appropriate.

Epilepsy and pregnancy

The patient must be advised about teratogenicity of anti-convulsants before embarking on a pregnancy. Of the anticonvulsants, only lamotrigine may be free of terato-genic effects. Phenytoin and phenobarbitone cause cleft palate and hare lip. Carbamazepine and sodium valproate cause spina bifida. The adverse effects of carbamazepine and sodium valproate can be reduced if the mother takes folic acid (5 mg daily) before conception and during the first 3 months of the pregnancy. It is unwise to withdraw anticonvulsants because of a planned pregnancy or once conception is known for certain to have occurred.

Epilepsy and the oral contraceptive

Many of the anticonvulsants (including phenobarbitone, primidone, carbamazepine and topiramate) induce liver enzymes and accelerate the metabolism of the oral contra-ceptive. Patients should take a combined oral contraceptive pill that contains 50 μg of oestrogen.

Drug levels

Drug levels are performed too frequently both in hospital and general practice. They are principally of use in manag-ing the dosage of phenytoin, since dosage–serum level relationships for phenytoin are not linear (Figure 8). Otherwise, the main value of drug levels is to check patient compliance. If drug levels are taken, their timing and rela-tionship to dosage should be recorded. It is interesting to note that analysis of general practice activity suggests that sodium valproate levels are requested as often as pheny-toin levels.[26]

Adequate record-keeping

Essential to good-quality epilepsy care are meticulous records that document previous investigations, previous

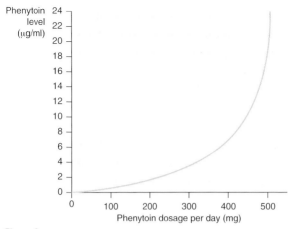

Figure 8
Phenytoin serum levels according to daily dosage in one patient

drug exposure and adverse events. In one general practice survey, the reason for withdrawal of previously prescribed anticonvulsants was recorded in only 64 per cent of cases.[26] If changes to drug regimens are to be made, it is probably wise to add on the new drug before contemplating withdrawal of existing therapy. Polypharmacy, certainly with more than two drugs, is to be avoided.

Deteriorating control

A surprisingly large number of patients with epilepsy are non-compliant with their medication. If non-compliance is a problem, a change to a drug that can be given once a day (e.g. phenytoin, lamotrigine, valproate retard) may enhance compliance. Alcohol abuse can exacerbate epilepsy, either by lowering seizure threshold or by interfering with the metabolism of anticonvulsant medication.

Improving care

It has been suggested that epilepsy management would be enhanced by providing structured care, implying the operation of a disease register, a prescription register and a recall system.[27] Younger patients and those who belong to self-help groups tend to have a greater knowledge of their epilepsy. Patients' understanding may be enhanced by utilizing a specialist nurse.[26]

Practice points

- Regular review of patients with epilepsy should be the aim
- Poor compliance and alcohol abuse are the most likely causes of deteriorating control
- Multiple drug therapy is best avoided

Common fallacies

- That patients with minor epileptic events do not need advice about driving
- That once anticonvulsant therapy has been initiated, it must be continued on a life-long basis
- That response to an anticonvulsant occurs only if the serum level of the drug is in the 'therapeutic' range

Parkinson's disease

Epidemiology

The incidence rate of Parkinson's disease was estimated as 19 per 100,000 per year in the United Kingdom Surveillance Study.[3] Parkinsonism was thought to be responsible for 20 consultations per year in a practice of 10,000 in Fry's data.[2] It accounts for 1.9 per cent of new neurology outpatient referrals.[4] It has been estimated that there will be three or four patients with Parkinson's disease on an average general practice list.[29] The condition is therefore common, and it will become more so over the next 20 years as the population ages.

It is vital, when appraising the condition, to separate it from those conditions that mimic the appearance of Parkinson's disease but that are due to another underlying pathology. Some of these conditions (e.g. multisystem atrophy, progressive supranuclear palsy) are rare. Drug-induced parkinsonism, on the other hand, is common and frequently overlooked. Drug-induced parkinsonism tends to be symmetrical and to cause a predominant akinetic–rigid syndrome, tremor being much less likely. The problem can persist for months after withdrawal of neuroleptic medication. It accounted for 18 per cent of patients who had been given a putative diagnosis of Parkinson's disease in one population survey.[29]

Specific issues

Is it Parkinson's disease?

Tremor is present at the time of onset of Parkinson's disease in about two-thirds of patients. Typically it is a rest tremor that disappears briefly during movement. A pill-rolling tremor is uncommon; more characteristic are flexion–extension movements of the fingers or wrist or a pronator–supinator movement of the forearm. The tremor may well be confined to one side.

A faster, postural tremor can also occur in Parkinson's disease. If the tremor is postural rather than resting, consider the possibility of an essential tremor syndrome. Such a tremor tends to run in families and is relieved by alcohol in about 50 per cent of cases.

In Parkinson's disease, there is likely to be some rigidity, and paucity of movement, though these changes may be mild (Figure 9). Watch the patient walking. Typically there is a reduction of arm swing on the affected side. Ask the patient about writing, and look at the patient's script. Rigidity may declare itself indirectly (e.g. in the form of a frozen shoulder).

Check the drug history. Several drugs other than the neuroleptics have been incriminated as causing an akinetic–rigid syndrome (Table 11).

Should the patient be referred?

There are no particular investigations for Parkinson's disease, though imaging is sometimes performed to exclude conditions that can mimic the disease. Referral is partly based on the general practitioner's confidence in the diag-

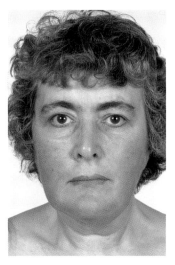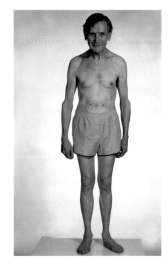

Figure 9
Facial appearance and mild kyphotic posture in two patients with early Parkinson's Disease

Presynaptic dopamine depletors (reserpine, tetrabenazine)

Neuroleptics (butyrophenones, phenothiazines, thioxantines)

Antiemetics (metoclopramide)

Calcium antagonists (cinnarizine, flunarizine, amlodipine (?), diltiazem (?))

Indomethacin

Cyclosporin

Valproate

Lithium (rarely)

Table 11
Drug-induced parkinsonism

nosis and partly on the patient's wishes. At this early stage, the patient is not likely to start medication but will probably simply be seen again at a later stage to assess the tempo of the disease and the accuracy of its diagnosis.

Established Parkinson's disease

With a firm diagnosis of Parkinson's disease and the patient stabilized on therapy (which may be a slow-release form of levodopa or a dopaminergic agonist), follow-up can reasonably rest with the general practitioner in the early stages of the disease if the drug is well tolerated. If nausea is a problem, the drug should be taken after food rather than before it. Absorption of levodopa can be hindered by taking meals high in protein. The patient should be advised to have regular meals of roughly equal size.

Review at 6-monthly intervals is reasonable. Ways of assessing benefit include:

- looking at samples of the patient's handwriting;

- checking the patient's walking speed;

- checking the patient's ability to stand from the sitting position without using the upper limbs.

Decline in benefit from therapy

After some 5–7 years, patients begin to show a decline in benefit. Their response to medication may fluctuate, and involuntary movements, typically choreiform or dystonic, start to emerge. Re-referral at this stage is appropriate.

Options that will be considered include increasing the frequency of dosing, adding an agonist to the regime (e.g. pergolide, ropinirole, cabergoline, pramipexole) or adding entacapone, a drug that inhibits peripheral breakdown of Dopa and so enhances its central effects.

Later problems

Increasing confusion

A major problem in the later stages of Parkinson's disease is an episodic confusional state interspersed with hallucinations. The condition is helped by a dosage reduction of levodopa but at the potential cost of exacerbating the disease. Quetiapine appears to be the best choice for controlling such symptoms with the least chance of exacerbating the Parkinson's disease.

Dementia

Dementia is more common in Parkinson's disease than was originally recognized. It affects about one in six patients. Its appearance is likely to result in greater intolerance of the anti-Parkinsonian drugs.

Freezing attacks

As the disease advances, freezing episodes emerge in which the patient unexpectedly freezes into immobility. The episodes last about 30 minutes and often occur several times a day. During a freezing attack the patient may be virtually incapable of movement. The attacks respond to subcutaneous apomorphine and need to be assessed by the hospital service.

The overall problem

Patients should be encouraged to join the Parkinson's Disease Society. It has been suggested that the input of a specialist nurse can be invaluable in co-ordinating care, recognizing problems at an early stage and liaising with various aspects of the social services.[6]

Practice points

- Make a careful check for recent drug exposure when a patient presents with apparent Parkinson's disease

- Offer periodic practice reviews for the parkinsonian patient, even if the patient apparently is well controlled

- Try to anticipate the later complications of the disease, and the need for input from the social services

Common fallacies

- That a marked asymmetry of signs makes idiopathic Parkinson's disease unlikely

- That treatment must be initiated immediately if a diagnosis of Parkinson's disease has been made

- That any drug-induced effect can be discounted if the drug was withdrawn more than one month ago

Dementia

Epidemiology

Only presenile dementia was included in the UK General Practice Survey already referred to.[3] The age- and sex-adjusted incidence rate was calculated to be 4 per 100,000. In unselected neurology outpatient practice, dementia accounts for 1.5 per cent of referrals. The prevalence of dementia rises with age and reaches 20 per cent or more in those aged over 80. With the projection of an increasingly ageing population in the UK (estimated to peak about 2025), the extent of the problem will inevitably grow.[30] On average, a general practitioner will have about 15 patients with dementia on the list. At least one-quarter of general practitioners feel uneasy about making the diagnosis.[31] Although most cases of dementia are recognized, assessment of cognitive status in general practice is as likely to be based on interview as on formal tests of cognition.[32]

Specific issues

Raising one's suspicion

Patients with early dementia are almost invariably accompanied by a relative, since it is the relative's concern, rather than the patient's, that has triggered the consultation.[33] Suggestive symptoms include memory impairment, a loss of initiative and drive and unexplained behaviour. If the patient is still working, changes in work performance are likely to have been noted.

Is it depression?

Many patients with dementia develop a depressive illness, and many patients with a primary depressive illness may show features that suggest a dementing process.

Features that suggest depression rather than dementia include:[34]

- Relatively short duration of symptoms
- Substantial complaints made by the patient rather than by a relative
- Apparent distress caused by the memory dysfunction
- Equal effects on recent and long-term memory

How best to screen for dementia in general practice

Assessments of dementia based on unstructured interviews alone are fraught with error. In one general practice survey, 15 patients previously labelled as demented (14 possibly and one definite) were rated as not demented when assessed on an information–orientation scale.[35] They included one patient with dysphasia, two with deafness, six with depression and three with extreme frailty.

Attempts have been made to determine which screening test is of most value in a general practice setting, and the Mini-Mental State Examination has been found to be the most appropriate.[36] This test can be administered in 5 minutes and it is well-known and its limitations are well recognized (Table 12).

Orientation

1. What is the year, season, date, month, day? (One point for each correct answer.)
2. Where are we? Country, county, town, hospital, floor? (One point for each correct answer.)

Registration

3. Name three objects taking 1 s to say each. Then ask the patient to repeat them. One point for each correct answer. Repeat the questions until the patient learns all three.

Attention and calculation

4. Serial sevens. One point for each correct answer. Stop after five answers. Alternative, spell 'world' backwards.

Recall

5. Ask for the names of the three objects asked in Question 3. One point for each correct answer.

Language

6. Point to a pencil and a watch. Have the patient name them for you. One point for each answer.
7. Have the patient repeat 'No, ifs, ands or buts.' One point.
8. Have the patient follow a three-stage command: 'Take the paper in your right hand, fold the paper in half, put the paper on the floor.' Three points
9. Have the patient read and obey the following: Close your eyes. (Write this in large letters.) One point.
10. Have the patient write a sentence of his or her own choice. (The sentence must contain a subject and an object and make some sense.) Ignore spelling errors when scoring. One point.
11. Have the patient draw two intersecting pentagons with equal sides. Give one point if all the sides and angles are preserved and if the intersecting sides form a quadrangle.

Maximum score = 30 points

Table 12
The Mini-Mental State Examination

When to refer

If the diagnosis of dementia appears likely (based on a screening appraisal and the elimination of a pseudode-mentia caused by depression) referral is reasonable. The referral may be to a psychiatrist, a neurologist or to a geri-atrician, according to local availability. The patient will then receive a more in-depth assessment and will have appro-priate blood tests and some form of imaging. These tests are designed to identify so-called reversible forms of dementia, such as:

- hypothyroidism;

- vitamin B_{12} deficiency;

- intracranial tumour.

The diagnosis may be of dementia of Alzheimer-type or related to vascular disease or of dementia for which the pathological basis remains uncertain.

Management of the established condition

It is apparent that many general practitioners (60 per cent in one series) are reluctant to disclose the diagnosis of dementia to their patients.[32] Informed discussion is essen-tial, however, both in terms of planning care, and in terms of using drug therapy. At present, drug intervention is of limited value. Both donepezil and rivastigmine show a symptomatic benefit that can last for several months. Areas that show benefit include activities of daily living and global functioning.

The later stages

The physical and emotional burden posed by dementia patients on their carers is profound. Despite this, many such patients stay within the family unit for some years.

Patients with a known diagnosis of dementia should be assessed at home at regular intervals. Appropriate social services can be introduced, respite care organized, and planning for inpatient care done in collaboration with the family.

Practice points

- It is essential to recognize a depressive illness masquerading as dementia

- A brief mental assessment such as the Mini-Mental State Examination can be rapidly administered and provide a baseline measure of cognitive function

- A history from a relative is of major value when appraising a patient for possible dementia

Common fallacies

- That patients with a communication disorder are likely to be demented

- That dementia is a likely diagnosis in a younger patient complaining of memory loss

- That screening for dementia is not feasible in a general practice setting

References

1. Jerrett WA. Headaches in general practice, *The Practitioner* (1979) **222**: 549–55.

2. Fry J, Sandler G. *Common Diseases. Their Nature, Presentation and Care*, 5th edn. Dordrecht, Boston, London: Kluwer Academic Publishers (1993).

3. MacDonald BK, Cockerell OC, Sander JWAS et al. The incidence and lifetime prevalence of neurological disorders in a prospective community-based study in the UK. *Brain* (2000) **123**: 665–76.

4. Perkin GD. An analysis of 7836 successive new outpatient referrals. *J Neurol Neurosurg Psychiatry* (1989) **52**: 447–8.

5. Ebrahim S. Changing patterns of consultation in general practice: fourth national morbidity study, 1991–1992. *Br J Gen Pract* (1995) **45**: 283–5.

6. Henry S. Wanted. 240 Parkinson's disease nurse specialists. *Geriatr Med* (2000) **30**: 19–20.

7. Collie DA, Sellar RJ, Steyn JP, Cull RE. The diagnostic yield of magnetic resonance imaging (MRI) of the brain and spine requested by general practitioners: comparison with hospital clinicians. *Br J Gen Pract* (1999) **49**: 559–61.

8. Milne JS. Headache in general practice. *Scot Med J* (1965) **10**: 251–3.

9. Perkin GD. *Basic Neurology* (Chichester: Ellis Horwood Limited, 1986).

10. Yardley L, Owen N, Nazareth I, Luxon L. Prevalence and presentation of dizziness in a general practice community sample of working age people. *Br J Gen Pract* (1998) **48**: 1131–5.

11. Bird JC, Beynon GJ, Prevost AT, Baguley DM. An analysis of referral patterns for dizziness in the primary care setting. *Br J Gen Pract* (1998) **48**: 1828–32.

12. Yardley L, Beech S, Zander L et al. A randomized controlled trial of exercise therapy for dizziness and vertigo in primary care, *Br J Gen Pract* (1998) **48**: 1136–40.

13. Foster CA, Baloh RW. Episode vertigo. In Bakel RE (ed). *Conn's current therapy*. Philadelphia: Saunders 1995: 839.

14. MacLennan WJ. Confusion: the cause is the key. *Practitioner* (1999) **243**: 209–13.

15. Casey DA, De Fazio JV Jr, Van Sickle K, Lippmann SB. Delirium: quick recognition, careful evaluation and appropriate treatment. *Postgrad Med* (1996) **100**: 121–34.

16. Brockenhurst JC, Morris P, Andrews K et al. Social effects of stroke. *Soc Sci Med* (1981) **15A**: 35–39.

17. Cassidy TP, Gray CS. Stroke and the carer. *Br J Gen Pract* (1991) **41**: 267–8.

18. Ebrahim S, Nouri F. Caring for stroke patients at home. *Int Rehabil Med* (1986) **8**: 171–3.

19. Murphy E. Social origins of depression in old age. *Br J Psychiatry* (1982) **141**: 135–42.

20. Kinsella GJ, Duffy FD. Psychosocial readjustment in spouses of aphasic patients. *Scand J Rehabil Med* (1979) **11**: 129–32.

21. Steiner TJ, MacGregor EA, Davies PTG. *Guidelines for All Doctors in the Diagnosis and Management of Migraine and Tension-Type Headache*. (London: 1999 British Association for the Study of Headache, Charing Cross Hospital, London W6 8RF).

22. Goodridge G, Shorvon SD. Epileptic seizures in a population of 6000. 1: Demography, diagnosis and classification, and the role of the Hospital services. *BMJ* (1983) **287**: 641–4.

23. Hopkins A, Scambler G. How doctors deal with epilepsy. *Lancet* (1977) **1**: 183–6.

24. Thapar AK. Care of patients with epilepsy in the community: will new initiatives address old problems? *Br J Gen Pract* (1996) **46**: 37–42.

25. Ridsdale L, Jeffery S, Robins D et al. Epilepsy monitoring and advice recorded: general practitioners' views, current practice and patients' preferences. *Br J Gen Pract* (1966) **46**: 11–14.

26. Jacoby A, Graham-Jones S, Baker G et al. A general practice records audit of the process of care for people with epilepsy. *Br J Gen Pract* (1996) **46**: 595–9.

27. White P. Structured management in primary care of patients with epilepsy. *Br J Gen Pract* (1996) **46**: 3.

28. Ridsdale L, Kwan I, Cryer C. The effect of a special nurse on patients' knowledge of epilepsy and their emotional state. *Br J Gen Pract* (1999) **49**: 285–9.

29. Mutch WJ, Dingwall-Fordyce I, Downie AW et al. Parkinson's disease in a Scottish city. *BMJ* (1986) **292**: 534–6.

30. Perkin GD. The likely impact of demographic changes on the incidence and prevalence of neurological disease: demography in the United Kingdom. *J Neurol Neurosurg Psychiatry* (1997) **63 (Suppl 1)**: S8–S10.

31. Vassilas CA, Donaldson J. Telling the truth: what do general practitioners say to patients with dementia or terminal cancer? *Br J Gen Pract* (1998) **48**: 1081–2.

32. O'Connor DW, Pollitt PA, Hyde JB et al. Do general practitioners miss dementia in elderly patients? *BMJ* (1988) **297**: 1107–10.

33. Kennedy A, Rossor M. Management of dementia. *Practitioner* (1993) **237**: 103–7.

34. Daoud JB. Memory loss. *Update* (8 July 1998) 62–5.

35. O'Connor DW, Fertig A, Grande MJ et al. Dementia in general practice: the practical consequences of a more positive approach to diagnosis. *Br J Gen Pract* (1993) **43**: 185–8.

36. Wilcock GK, Ashworth DL, Langfield JA et al. Detecting patients with Alzheimer's disease suitable for drug treatment: comparison of three methods of assessment. *Br J Gen Pract* (1994) **44**:

Index